Lyme Disease -
What You Need to Know

Cause, Symptoms and Treatment for This Often Mis-Diagnosed Disease

RON KNESS

Contents

Disclaimer

This publication is for informational purposes only and is not intended as medical advice. Medical advice should always be obtained from a qualified medical professional for any health conditions or symptoms associated with them.
Every possible effort has been made in preparing and researching this material. We make no warranties with respect to the accuracy, applicability of its contents or any omissions.

See your healthcare professional before starting any diet, health or exercise program!

Introduction

Around 3 million people in the US are living with Lyme disease, with about 300,000 new cases each year. Lyme diseases is highly treatable if caught early. However, if it is not caught early, it can lead to various health issues and become a chronic problem that will cause a range of symptoms.

In this guide you will learn the essentials about Lyme disease, what it is, how to treat it, and above all, how to prevent it. Let's get started with what Lyme Disease (LD) is and where it comes from.

What Is Lyme Disease?

Lyme disease is an infectious disease caused by a bacterium called Borrelia burgdorferi. The bacteria are transmitted to humans through the bite of infected black-legged ticks, also known as a deer tick. The bite introduces the bacteria into the bloodstream of the victim. It is therefore common in areas which have deer.

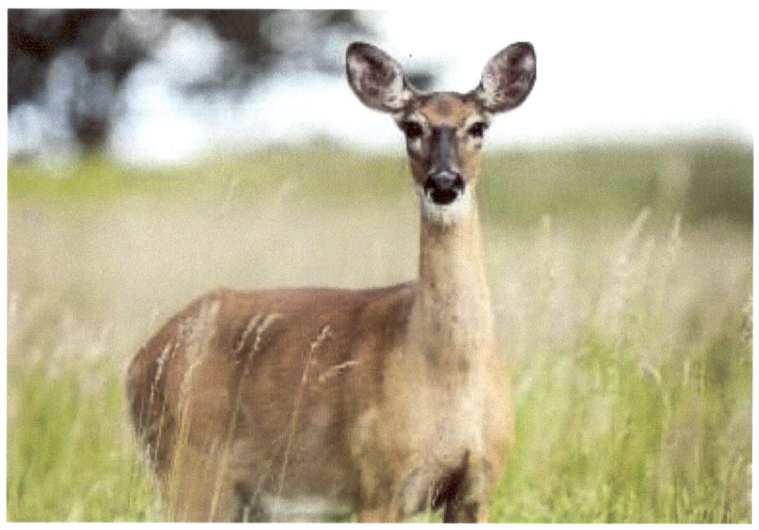

Lyme disease may present at first like the flu, with:

- Fever
- Headache
- Fatigue/tiredness even after resting
- Aches and pains

The most common sign of having been bitten by a tick infected with LD is a bullseye rash, that is, a red spot with a white and then an outer red ring around it.

It was first referred to in the 1970s as Lyme arthritis, which will give you an idea of the most common symptoms.

LD is generally not harmful if it is caught early. However, if left untreated, the infection can spread to the:

- Joints
- Heart
- Nervous system

... leading to a range of symptoms depending on how advanced the progress of the infection.

The bacteria are a spirochete, that is, a spiral-shaped bacterium that resembles a corkscrew. Another example of a spirochete would be the syphilis virus. Spirochetes can be difficult to treat, so prevention or early detection are best for successfully dealing with LD.

So, what are ticks? And does all tick carry LD? Let's look at these questions in the next chapter.

How Is Lyme Disease Contracted?

Ticks are small, hard-shelled insects that are related to spiders. They are parasites that live on the blood of mammals, and sometimes even reptiles and amphibians.

Lyme disease is a tick-borne disease caused by bacteria belonging to the genus Borrelia transmitted through the bite of infected ticks belonging to the genus Ixodes, and in particular, Ixodes scapularis, the black-legged tick, also known as the deer tick.

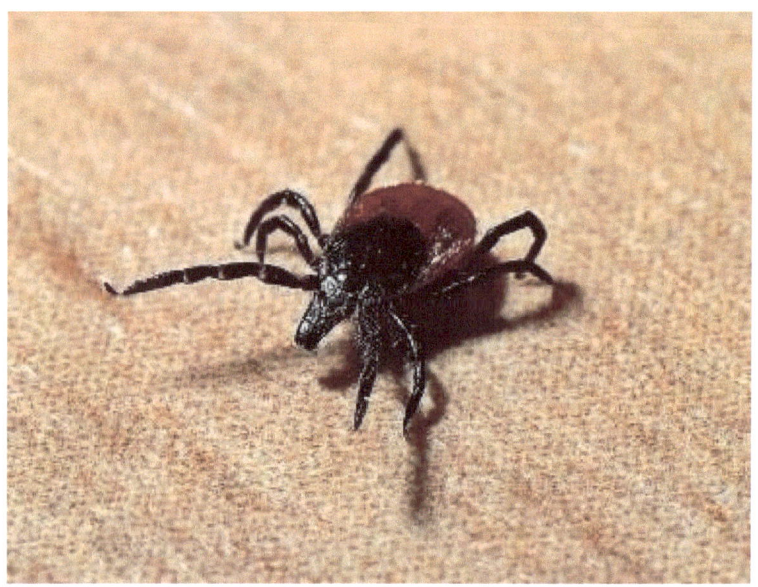

Of the different types in the genus Borrelia, Borrelia burgdorferi is the predominant bacteria that cause illness in North America. However, another type called Borrelia mayonii has recently been discovered as a cause of Lyme disease in the upper Midwestern United States.

It has been found in blacklegged ticks (Ixodes scapularis) in Minnesota and Wisconsin.

Borrelia miyamotoi infection has also recently been described as a cause of illness in the US, with some patients showing Lyme-like symptoms and others the symptoms of other tickborne diseases. Two other types - Borrelia afzelii and Borrelia garinii - are the main causes of Lyme in Europe and Asia. Symptoms vary amongst the different strains.

Ticks can move from host to host. They become infected when they feed on deer, birds, and rodents, who are reservoirs for the bacteria and spread it to humans. The spread is typically caused by nymphs, or young, immature ticks, which are harder to detect than a full-grown adult. The ticks bite and engorge with blood. The tick mouthparts introduce the bacteria into the bloodstream.

Ticks like shady, wooded areas and grass. Due to global warming, tick populations appear to be moving further north in latitude, preferring cooler weather. Lyme disease is mostly found in the Northeastern part of the United States. It is named after the town of Lyme, Connecticut, which was the 'ground zero' for the discovery of the illness.
However, around 80 countries around the world have reported cases. If there are deer around, there are deer ticks, and thus a danger of Lyme disease.

In the Pacific Northwest, the main carrier is the Western black-legged tick. In the south, cases have been reported in relation to the Lone Star tick.

Learning to identify ticks can be one of the best ways to know how to treat any symptoms that might arise after being out in the woods or exposed to certain animals. View this chart at: http://www.tickencounter.org/tick_identification/tickid_nonflash

Preventing tick bites on yourself, and infestation on any companion animals, such as dogs or cats that go outside, can help prevent LD. In particular, if you have a long-haired animal, it is very easy for a tick to attach itself to your pet. If you sleep with your pet, the tick could transfer to you.

A good flea and tick treatment such as Frontline, plus a tick collar if you live in the North and/or your pets spend a lot of time outside, can stop ticks in their tracks. They need to be renewed every month.

Other insects
Ticks are not the only insects that can carry Lyme disease. It can also be transmitted and carried by:
- Mosquitoes
- Spiders
- Mites
- Lice

But the majority of infections are tick-related. To learn more, see "Why is Lyme Disease-not just tick-borne anymore?" http://www.care2.com/greenliving/why-is-lyme-disease-not-just-tick-borne-anymore.html

Now that you know where LD comes from and how it is contracted, let's look at the symptoms of LD.

What Are the Symptoms of Lyme Disease?

The symptoms of LD vary depending on the stage of the illness and the strain of the bacteria.

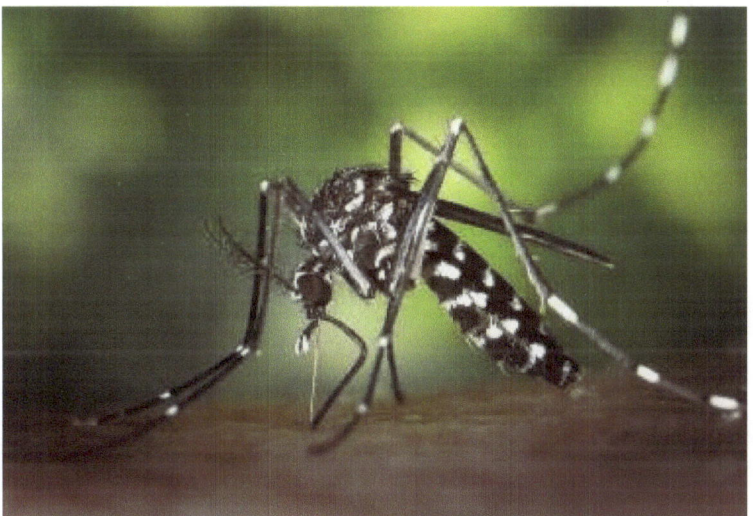

Acute Symptoms

As noted earlier, the most common strain of bacteria is Borrelia burgdorferi. Common symptoms from this strain of tick includes:

- fever
- headache
- fatigue/tiredness even after resting
- swollen lymph nodes
- aches and pains

This strain of bacteria produces the 'bullseye rash', that is, a red spot with a white and then an outer red ring around it.

This usually helps to distinguish it from other tick-borne diseases, of which there are many.

A blood test is often used to diagnose LD. However, there are a lot of 'false positives' with the test that can lead to over-diagnosis or misdiagnosis.

Generally speaking, if a person spends a lot of time outdoors in wooden areas and in cool areas with tall grass, and starts experiencing symptoms noted, they should get checked by a doctor.

In some cases, a patient can experience Bell's Palsy. This is a sudden paralysis of one of the facial nerves. It is often mistaken for stroke because it comes on suddenly and causes the face to droop and this can cause the person to have trouble speaking.

Bell's palsy is connected with LD, shingles and other viral infections. In most cases, antibiotics will resolve it within a couple of months, but other people will experience long-term paralysis or muscle weakness.

Borrelia mayonii

This strain of Lyme disease was discovered by doctors at the Mayo Clinic in Minnesota in 2016. They have reported the following symptoms:

- nausea
- vomiting
- widespread rash
- unusually high levels of spirochetes in the blood

Two strains of bacteria are responsible for almost 100% of the cases in Europe - Borrelia afzelii and Borrelia garinii.

Borrelia afzelii

This appears in 85% of bullseye rashes in Europe. The symptoms are the same as those of North American Lyme. Many of its symptoms are related to the skin.
https://microbewiki.kenyon.edu/index.php/Borrelia_afzelii

Borrelia garinii

This accounts for 15% of cases of bullseye rashes in Europe. It causes various skin manifestations and can affect the brain with what is termed white matter encephalitis, that is, swelling and possible damage to the brain, and headache. The pain can be so severe that some patients are tested for the brain infection meningitis.

Borrelia miyamotoi (Asia and North America)

This strain will present with LD rash in less than 10% of cases. The strain was discovered in Japan in the 1990s but is now present in 2 different species of ticks in the US, including the deer tick. The symptoms can be similar to LD or to a couple of other tick-borne illnesses, such as anaplasmosis or tick-borne relapsing fever. The Annals of Internal Medicine reported recently that this strain of bacteria is more widespread than previously thought.
http://annals.org/aim/article/2301402/borrelia-miyamotoi-disease-northeastern-united-states-case-series

Some tickborne diseases have similar symptoms. We will look later in this guide at illnesses that can be mistaken for Lyme Disease.

Chronic Lyme Disease

Chronic Lyme disease, or CLD, is also referred to second or third stage Lyme disease, or post-treatment Lyme disease (PTLD). Not all the bacteria have been destroyed, and the spirochetes have penetrated and hidden themselves in tissue in one or more parts of the body where they can cause a range of issues.

Symptoms

The most common symptoms are:
- arthritis, rheumatological symptoms
- aches, pains, joint pain,
- headaches, brain and spine inflammation, neurological issues
- irregular heartbeat, slow or fast heart beat
- bullseye rash
- ophthalmological issues

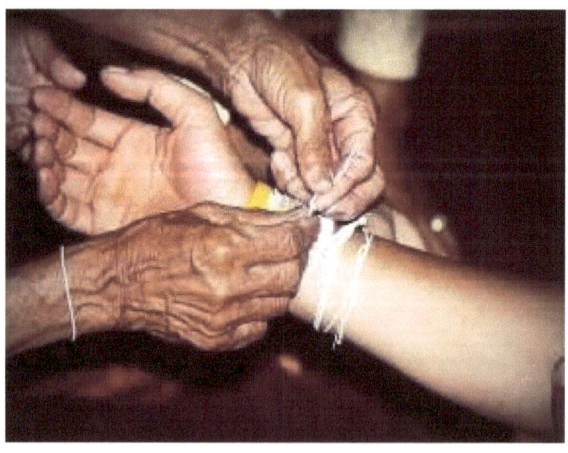

Arthritis, rheumatological symptoms

Aches, pains, joint pain, inflammation, with the joint feeling hot or as though they are on fire.

Headaches, brain and spine inflammation, neurological issues

Sometimes the symptoms are so severe that the patient is tested for meningitis. It can also include Bell's palsy-this can lead to facial paralysis on one side of the face for 1 to several months. In rare cases, it can be permanent.

Irregular heartbeat, slow or fast heart beat (tachycardia or bradycardia).

This can be cause by Lyme carditis, an infection of the heart muscle that can be serious and in some cases fatal because it can lead to sudden cardiac arrest and death. In many cases, it will be treated with a pacemaker, or sometimes an implanted defibrillator, to keep the heart beating at a regular rate.

Bullseye rash - this can appear at the site of the bite, but it can also result in more than one lesion on any part of the body. There are not usually any dermatologic symptoms such as itchiness or soreness, though the rash can be very red and inflamed looking. The spots will often appear when symptoms are most severe.

Ophthalmological issues

Lyme can cause a range of symptoms, from pink eye (conjunctivitis), dry eye, and other eye problems.

Women report getting bullseyes during their periods and their symptoms worsening in general, which might perhaps indicate the body is put under even more stress at these times of the month.

Lyme disease can sometimes be a tricky disease to treat if it is not spotted early. It can also be mistaken for a number of different conditions. Let's look at a couple of the main ones in the next chapter.

Other Disorders Frequently Misdiagnosed as Lyme Disease

Lyme disease presents with a range of symptoms that are similar to that of the flu or a viral infection. Only around 70% to 80% of people get the bullseye rash, which means those who don't might have their symptoms mistaken for other illnesses.

For example, tiredness all the time can be taken for chronic fatigue syndrome. Aches and pains can be mistaken for arthritis or fibromyalgia. The inflammation is often mistaken for autoimmune disorders, in which the body starts to attack itself, such as rheumatoid arthritis or multiple sclerosis.

There are quite a few tickborne diseases that can also be similar to that of Lyme disease. For example, several illnesses, including possibly Lyme, are connected with the Borrelia miyamotoi strain of bacteria. One of the illnesses is termed Borrelia miyamotoi Disease, or BMD.

Typical symptoms include:
- fever
- aches and pains
- flu-like symptoms

- headache and
- sometimes rash

In some cases, the doctors might think this is anaplasmosis infection based on blood tests which show abnormal cells. In about 50% of cases, patients were thought to have a severe infection known as sepsis, and about 25% ended up in the hospital because their symptoms were so severe. In some cases, the Lyme-like symptoms were so severe that they were mistaken for meningitis.

Borrelia miyamotoi can also carry tickborne relapsing fever. TRF is similar to Lyme, but the key word is relapsing, that is, seeming to get better, but then becoming sick again. Signs to look out for include:

- high fever (e.g., 103° F)
- headache
- muscle pain
- aching joints

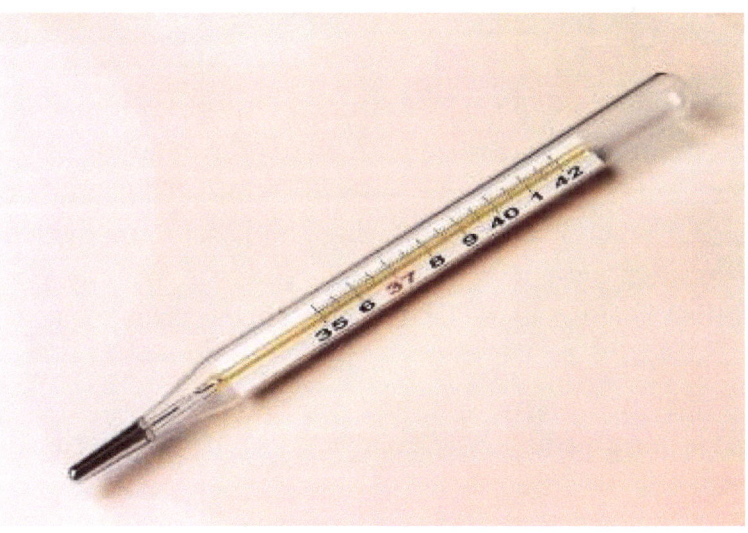

Symptoms will develop about a week after being bitten. The person will get sick for 3 days, seem better for 7, get sick again for 3 days, and so on. Without antibiotics, this cycle can repeat over and over again for many months.

Rocky Mountain Spotted Fever?

Rocky Mountain Spotted Fever, commonly abbreviated as RMSF, is an infectious disease carried by various ticks, which bite a person and infect them with rickettsia group bacteria.

About 20,000 cases occur in the US each year, mainly in the spring and summer months when people spend more time outdoors in the wild. Contrary to the name, RMSF is pretty rare, but can be fatal if it is not diagnosed and treated promptly. A blood test can determine whether or a person has it, and the correct treatment started.

The sources of infection are tick-borne and carried by::
- RMSF tick
- American Dog tick
- Brown Dog tick

It can also be spread via feces from an infected animal or person coming into contact with an open wound, or eating food contaminated with the feces of an infected person or animal. For this reason, practicing good bathroom hygiene, such as always washing hands well, and food hygiene, including keeping food covered so no insects can get at it, is key.

If no running water is available, hand sanitizer is better than nothing.

Where can you contract RMSF?

The name RMSF can be misleading because it does not just occur in the Rocky Mountain region, but all over North and South America. It was first identified in Idaho in 1896 and in the Rocky Mountain region generally, has spread over the years to a wider and wider area and has been reported in a majority of the states in the US.

What are the symptoms of RMSF:

Symptoms to watch out for include:

- fever
- headache
- muscle ache
- the distinctive rash that gives it its name-it used to be referred to as 'black measles'
- the tick bite site might look black or encrusted.

The trouble is that most people are not even aware that they have been bitten by a tick until they start to experience symptoms. The rash takes several days to develop, so this means delay in seeking treatment. It is usually treated with antibiotics. If the case progresses untreated, symptoms can become increasingly severe, and include:

- pain in the abdomen, joints, or muscles
- flu-like symptoms, including fever, chills, aches and pains
- loss of appetite
- nausea
- vomiting
- rashes, spots, red or black

Other reported symptoms include:

- red eyes

- sensitivity to light
- painful headache
- a rash on the palms of the hands and/or soles of the feet

Treatments for RMSF

The first treatment for RMSF is antibiotics to kill the bacteria causing the illness. The most commonly used is doxycycline, usually for 7 to 14 days.

If the disease progresses, patients with severe infections may require hospitalization due to blood clotting disorders, low sodium/electrolytes that can cause heart issues and elevated liver enzymes. In some cases, the patient may experience respiratory or neurological symptoms, or kidney problems.

At risk patients

In general, the prognosis for RMSF can be good. However, it depends on how soon it is diagnosed. Those most at risk include:

- elderly patients
- males
- African-Americans
- Alcoholics
- patients with the blood disorder G6PD deficiency which causes hemolysis.

Long-term health implications

Patients who had a particularly severe infection requiring prolonged hospitalization may have long-term health problems because the bacteria infects the endothelial cells that line the blood vessels throughout the body.

The damage that occurs in the blood vessels causes a disease known as vasculitis.

Vasculitis can result in internal bleeding or clotting in the brain, vital organs, or extremities, leading to loss of circulation and death of the tissue, or death of the patient. The tissue death may result in amputations.

Most patients have a good outcome, however, and recover several days to months after infection.

The most sensible way to avoid RMSF is to use insect repellent and be vigilant about ticks on yourself or your pets. Now that we know what to look for in terms of how LD and related illnesses are contracted and what the symptoms are, let's have a look at conventional treatments for LD.

What is the Difference Between Early Lyme Disease and Chronic Lyme?

There are a number of key differences between early Lyme disease and chronic Lyme disease. Lyme is highly treatable in its early stages. However, the longer it remains untreated, the more likely it will turn into chronic Lyme disease.

Acute Lyme Disease (ALD)
Acute Lyme comes on suddenly and is very like the flu, so a lot of people may mistake it for this common illness. However, if you have been walking in the woods or been on vacation in a wooded area, or one with deer, or walking in tall grass with a skirt or shorts on, it is possible for a tick to latch onto you.

The tick will usually have to remain on you for at least 24 hours to transmit the bacteria which causes Lyme. Baby ticks, known as nymphs, are only the size of a poppy seed, and adult ticks only the size of a sesame seed, so it is easy to pick up a tick and never even notice.

Pets who spend a lot of time outside in the tall grass are also prone to picking up ticks, especially if they are long-haired. The tick can then transfer onto a human family member. Keeping up with flea and tick protection each month with Frontline or a similar product will usually be enough to keep your pet safe. However, if you live in the northeast where Lyme is most common, a tick collar will offer even more protection.

If you do develop flu symptoms and have spent a lot of time outdoors in the previous week, suspect Lyme and get checked by a doctor.

The most obvious sign of early Lyme is a bullseye rash comprised of a red center with a white ring around it and then a red outer ring. Unfortunately, it is only present in about 70% to 80% of patients, leaving the others at risk of the disease progressing to chronic Lyme without them even knowing it.

Chronic Lyme Disease (CLD)
Chronic Lyme Disease can be a lot tougher to treat, and cause significant damage to one or more parts of the body. It can be described as a persistent infection due to the presence of the bacteria which causes Lyme, which is a spirochete. The corkscrew shape of spirochetes means they can attach onto tissue easily and are harder to get rid of. A more familiar spirochete is syphilis, and as history has shown, it is difficult to treat and has devastating long-term consequences, particularly neurological ones.

Neurological symptoms
Typical symptoms include:
- Frequent headaches/migraines that are not always relieved with painkillers
- A stiff neck
- Brain fog
- Memory loss
- Cognitive impairment to the point where doctors think it might be Alzheimer's or another form of dementia

- Nerve pain

Heart problems

Lyme carditis strikes at the heart muscle and can lead to various forms of damage and issues. It can make the heart beat slower (bradycardia) or faster (tachycardia) or irregularly. Experts compare a person who

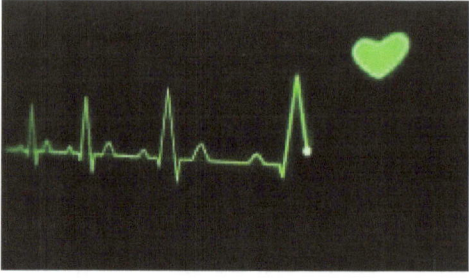

has Lyme carditis as having a similar quality of life to those with congestive heart failure. Heart failure will result in death if it is not managed properly with medications. A pacemaker might also be put in to help the heart work better, or a defibrillator to deal with rhythm issues.

Rheumatologic symptoms

Most people with chronic Lyme report aches and pains in the bones and joints, and in the muscles. The condition was once termed Lyme arthritis. The quality of life can be severely diminished due to the pain.

Treatment

Both ALD and CLD can be treated with antibiotics, though not always 100% successfully.

Now that you now the main differences between early Lyme disease and chronic Lyme disease, it might be time to check in with your doctor to start dealing with any symptoms you may have in a more proactive manner.

Conventional Treatment Options

Lyme disease is the result of a bacterial infection and is therefore highly treatable with antibiotics if caught early.

The CDC reports that the majority of people can make a complete recovery from Lyme disease after receiving a course of antibiotics for several weeks. The most common antibiotic treatment for Lyme infection is one or more 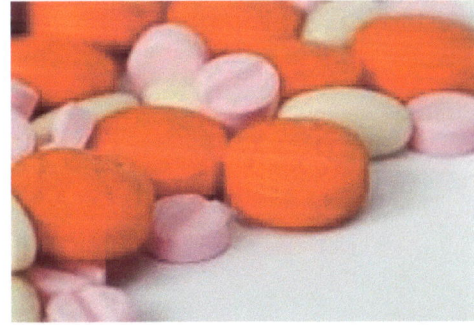 antibiotics, most often amoxicillin, cefuroxime axetil, and/or doxycycline, with the course lasting for 2 to 4 weeks. The decision will be based on symptoms and severity, and on allergies to any of these drugs.

In most cases, treatment will be successful, but if the infection spreads throughout the central nervous system, they will have lingering symptoms.

These drugs can also be a problem in pregnant women. Antibiotics can also produce their own set of symptoms, such as stomach issues, digestive issues and more.

If the LD is not caught early, it could progress to chronic disease, in which case, antibiotics may not be effective and run the risk of causing an imbalance in the body such that the LD actually start to thrive.

This being the case, it is important to take a holistic approach to treating LD to make the person with it as comfortable as possible and address symptoms without making them worse.

Let's look in the next chapter at the range of complementary and natural treatments that can be used in addition to traditional LD treatment.

Alternative Treatment Options

There are a number of complementary and natural approaches to LD that can offer relief from many of the more debilitating symptoms of Lyme.

There are several aspects to treatment which can work well together as a whole to maintain health and balance despite Lyme:

- Relieve pain
- Eat well
- Use supplements to support immune function
- Use natural remedies
- Avoid allergens
- Reduce stress
- Other treatment options

Let's look at each of these in turn.

Relieve Pain

LD can be very painful, from blinding headaches and paralyzing neck pain, to bones and joint aching and feeling as though they are 'on fire'. It might be tempting to take a lot of pain relievers such as aspirin and non-steroidal anti-inflammatory drugs (NSAIDS) such as Tylenol, but they can be hard on the stomach and carry a risk of side effects and even overdose.

Any natural pain relief methods can help. These can include:

Acupuncture and acupressure

Ancient Traditional Chinese Medicines (TCM) use the idea of meridians, or energy centers in the body, that need to be kept in balance, and can also be harnessed for health and healing. With acupuncture, small thin needles are used to stimulate the meridians using the pressure of the fingers or a knuckle. TCM will often use herbs as well to restore inner balance and relieve pain. In some cases, the herbs might even be burned and put on aching spots like a hot compress. Shiatsu is a similar healing modality that comes from Japan and also restores balance and heals pain.

Aromatherapy

Aromatherapy uses natural botanicals to relax and heal through the power of scent. The botanicals are called essential oils and each has its own particular effect. Some are even more powerful in combination. They can be inhaled in order to enhance mood and energy (such as citrus-based oils) or be relaxing and calming, such as lavender, rose and pine. These oils can also be used as part of massage.

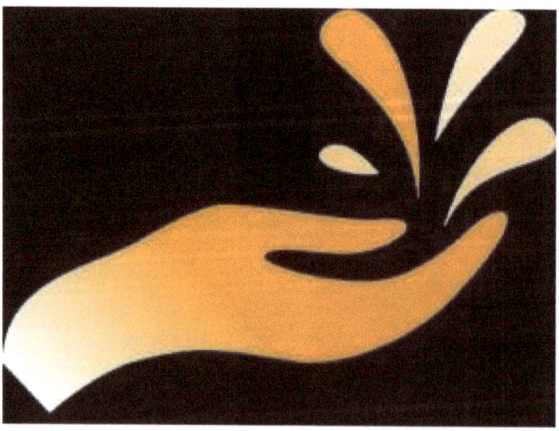

Massage Therapy

Massage is an effective natural pain relief method. You can learn how to massage yourself wherever you can manage to reach. You can also get a massage from your partner, or from a licensed massage therapist. Most insurance companies cover massage, acupressure and other complementary therapies these days, so check your coverage and see if one or more of these can offer effective pain relief.

Pain Relieving Creams

Some people find arthritis-related creams, such as those containing capsaicin, to offer relief on their bad days. Capsaicin comes from peppers. Don't apply to broken skin and keep away from the face and especially the eyes. Wash your hands well after using.

Eat well

LD is hard on the stomach and body in general. Antibiotics can make this worse. Therefore, it is important to eat right to maintain a healthy gut and get optimal nutrition.

An anti-inflammatory diet is the best option. You will avoid anything that has a lot of chemicals in it, such as convenience foods, and steer clear of sugar and salt. One of the best diets to follow is termed 'clean eating', consuming whole foods without a lot of preparation and ingredients, just simple, natural food.

This is also a good option because of what is termed leaky gut (read more about it here: **https://www.createspace.com/6528679**), in which the intestines are not able to absorb nutrition from your food properly and the broken-down food might actually leak out of your digestive tract and cause irritation and inflammation in the body.

Then we have antibiotics versus probiotics and prebiotics. Antibiotics are not able to discriminate and kill off both harmful and helpful bacteria alike. Probiotics, such as those found in yogurt, can restore the helpful bacteria. Prebiotics are what they probiotics feed on.

Good examples of probiotics include:

- Dark Chocolate
- Kefir-fermented goat's milk
- Miso Soup
- Pickles and pickled vegetables such as Italian giardiniera
- Sauerkraut
- Tempeh-fermented soy bean
- Yogurt

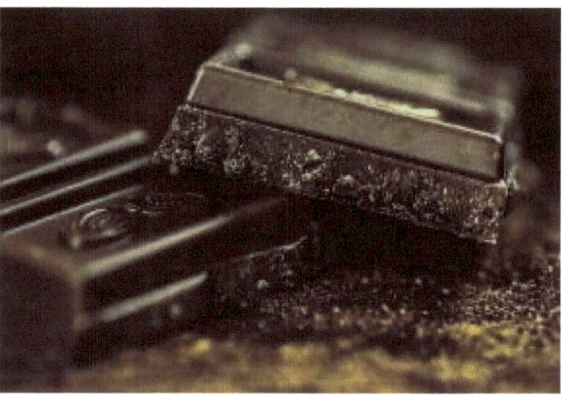

Good examples of prebiotics include:
- Asparagus
- Broccoli
- Brussels sprouts
- Cabbage
- Cauliflower
- Chicory (used as a coffee substitute)
- Collard greens
- Jerusalem artichokes
- Kale
- Leeks
- Onions

With so many delicious vegetables on this list, it's easy to eat healthy prebiotics.

One other really good food option is bone broth, that is, broth that has been made from animal bones cooked over a long period of time with a small amount of vinegar in order to get all of the vitamins and minerals out of the bones. It can be drunk as is, or used as a base for soups and stews.

Use vitamins and supplements to support immune function

There are a number of vitamins and minerals that can support your immune system to stop LD from getting the better of you. These include:

B vitamins
The B vitamins can't be stored in the body and are used up quickly, so replenishing them every day with whole grains and green leafy vegetables is essential.

If you smoke and/or are under a lot of stress, you will need even more.

CoQ10
This supplement supports the immune system and heart health.

Vitamin D
Fifteen minutes a day out in the sun (wear sunscreen) can help you produce all you need. Also, try dairy products and fortified soy products like soy milk to boost your immune system.

Calcium
Add calcium to your diet to support healthy immune function and bone and joint health.

Omega-3 fatty acids
These support the immune system and a healthy heart and brain, all of which can be affected by LD.

Magnesium and Zinc
These both support every function in the body, including maintaining good brain health.

Use natural herbal remedies

There are a number of herbs that can reduce inflammation and support balance in the body.

Cloves and Cinnamon
These two spices are great in smoothies or on top of a baked apple. They are also great with pumpkin, which is full of fiber.

Garlic
Eat fresh garlic regularly to ward off bacteria.

Ginger
Ginger root is delicious and a great natural antibiotic. Use in stir fries or drink as a tea.

Oregano
This is a staple ingredient in Italian food. Oregano has soothing, anti-inflammatory properties.

Marjoram
This leafy green herb has a nice lemony tang and is good in soups and stews.

Rosemary
Rosemary has outstanding anti-inflammatory and antibacterial properties. Use on chicken, sweet potatoes, or homemade roasted vegetables.

Sage and Thyme
These are both used to season soups, stews, and bread stuffing.

Turmeric
This bright yellow spice from India has been used for more than 5,000 years as a part of traditional medicine. It is perfect as an addition to any rice dish.

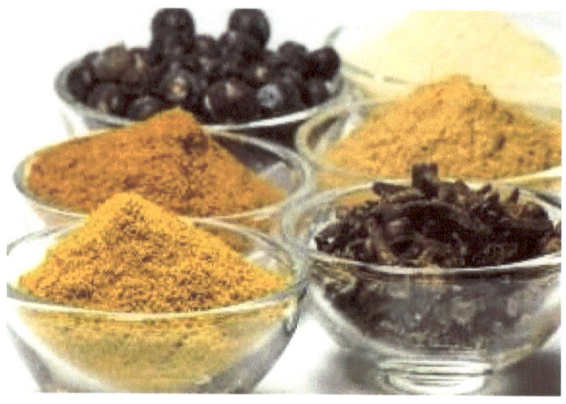

Avoid allergens

Steer clear of anything that makes you allergic, such as
pollen and ragweed. Avoid mold whenever possible. If you do
have seasonal allergies, try over the counter or natural
remedies. One natural remedy for hay fever is eating local
honey gathered within about a 10-mile radius of where you
live. You can usually find it at a farmer's market. Eat about 1
teaspoon per day; you can use it to sweeten your coffee or tea
as well, or as part of a fresh fruit and vegetable smoothie.

Reduce stress

Any long-term, chronic illness will take its toll if you don't
practice good self-care. Stress relief is essential for most
people in the modern world, but it can also relieve pain,
inflammation and 'brain fog' in people with LD. Learn more
about natural stress management and do things you enjoy
each day.

Meditation can help you relieve stress. Other options include
getting enough sleep, mindfulness practices, journaling,
visualization/guided imagery, and more.

Other treatment options

Rife generator/TENS unit
The Rife generator, or Transcutaneous Electrical Nerve Stimulation, stimulates health through various frequencies. The full list of all healing frequencies is here. http://www.royalrife.com/CAFL.pdf

You can make your own Rife machine for a fraction of what is being charged online. http://eternalspiralbooks.com/how-to-build-your-own-rife-machine-or-tens-unit/ Then record the frequencies and play them.

Note that with each treatment, you will become sicker before you become better. This is because the spirochetes release toxins into the blood when they die. The treatment protocol is usually doing it every day for 1 week and then resting for about 1 month. Use your other healing modalities and pain relief methods to cope with the worsening of symptoms after the treatment.

A warm bath or shower
A warm bath or shower can relax, relieve stress, and ease the aches and pains of LD. You can add essential oils to your bath for even more healing.

Meditation
Meditation can be a case of mind over matter if you use it to relieve your pain. It also improves mental clarity in order to combat the 'brain fog' that often comes with LD.

Detoxification

Detoxification helps remove any toxins in the body that might be causing health issues. A fast of 1 to 3 days of nothing but water and/or diluted fruit juice can help purge the system.

Detoxification of heavy metals

Our food chain has become so polluted that many dangerous heavy metals such as arsenic are now in the foods we eat. Beware of muscle milk, rice, and brown rice syrup in particular.

If you would like to do a heavy metal detox (which will also be a good general detox if you wish), eat:

- **Citrus and other fruits rich in vitamin C** - One humble kiwi has about 300% of your daily allowance. C supports skin and joint health and the immune system.

- **Spinach and kale** - They are not only packed with nutrition, they can help reduce the build-up of heavy metals like mercury in the body. If you eat canned tuna, only eat it twice a week, 3 days apart, to avoid dangerous mercury levels.

- **Garlic and onion** - These vegetables contain sulfur, which helps detox your liver from lead and arsenic.

- **Flax and chia seeds** - They have Omega-3 fats and cleanse the colon.

- **Fresh filtered water -** Drink eight 8-ounce glasses of water per day to flush out toxins.

- **Colloidal silver -** Colloidal silver used to be recommended by those with chronic LD, but the FDA and other agencies have determined that there is no supporting evidence that it can help with any illness. In addition, one of the most famous proponents of its use died at a relatively young age due to being poisoned by it. He was known as "Papa Smurf" or the blue man because the side effect of colloidal silver is to turn the skin blue. Stay safe and avoid this LD 'treatment'.

Exercise

Last, but by no means least, exercise relieves pain, boosts energy, and keeps the body healthy. It can be a great stress reliever as well.

To learn more about natural ways to treat LD, see: http://restormedicine.com/naturopathic-approaches-to-lyme-disease-treatment/

But even more important than learning how to treat LD is how to prevent it in the first place. Let's look at this topic in the next chapter.

Prevention Strategies

Thus, far we have discussed where LD comes from, what the symptoms are, and how to try to treat LD effectively depending on what stage of the illness you are at.

However, as with most health issues, prevention is the best strategy for dealing with it.

How to Prevent Tick and Insect Bites

When the spring and summer months arrive, the number of cases of LD increase. This is because people are spending more time outside in the nice weather. And as the grass grows higher, the ticks have an expanded habitat to lurk in. Add to this deer being more active, and their population increasing as new ones are born each spring, and you have a perfect storm of LD dangers to watch out for.

Fortunately, some forward planning and common sense can help you and your family stay safe when you are out in the woods, nature spots, or rustic places such as summer homes and cabins that are likely to be dark, cool, and an ideal hiding place for bugs.

The best way to prevent Lyme disease is to prevent tick bites outdoors and indoors. While you are outdoors, take the following precautionary steps:

- Avoid tall grass as much as possible.

- Wear long pants and long-sleeved shirts to minimize skin exposure to ticks.

- Don't run around the woods in shorts or a skirt.

- Tuck your pants into your socks to form a barrier to keep ticks out. They can very easily slip up a pant leg otherwise.

- Wear light-colored clothing so you can easily see ticks and other bugs.

- Check for ticks. They might be engorged with blood, in which case they will look plump and fat. Or they might not have eaten their fill yet, in which case they will look like a speck of dirt, a freckle or a 'skin tag'.

- Use effective tick repellents on your skin and/or on your clothing. When going outside, put on your sunscreen first. Wait until it dries. Then apply your repellent. Pay special attention to neck and ears.

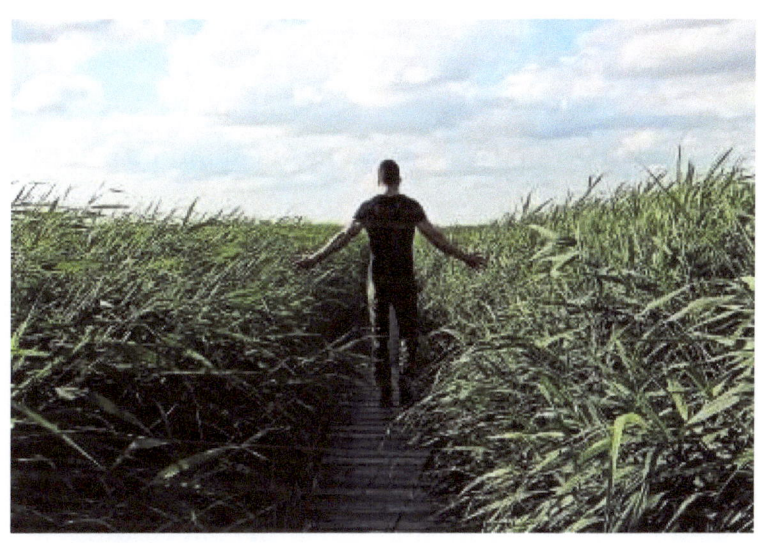

When you come indoors

Check your body for ticks, and check your children. Pay special attention to the head, armpits, and groin area. Remove any ticks promptly by following the instructions below.

Showering within a few hours of being outside can help remove any ticks and also avoid any skin reactions to your sunscreen and/or insect repellant.

Examine your gear and clothing to make sure no ticks have hitchhiked. Put your clothes in the dryer on high heat for an hour to kill any ticks.

Check your dog and pets for ticks each day.

Which is the right insect repellent for me and my family? Choose repellents that are registered by the Environmental Protection Agency (EPA). They have been evaluated for safety and effectiveness. Look for the EPA number on the label.

Read the label carefully for information about proper use, especially in reference to re-applying after swimming, in high heat when you are sweating, and so on.

DEET (N,N-diethyl-meta-toluamide) is effective against ticks and has been used safely for many years. Note that a higher percentage of DEET in a repellent does not mean that the protection is better, only that it tends to last longer and not need to be re-applied as often. DEET should not be used on infants younger than 2 months old or in concentrations greater than 30%.

Other repellents that may be effective against ticks include Picaridin (KBR 3023). This is derived from the oil of lemon eucalyptus and is therefore a more natural repellent.

For use on clothing:
Permethrin is an insecticide and insect repellent that can be used on clothing, shoes, bed nets, camping gear, back packs and more, to avoid 'hitchhikers' of all kinds, including ticks. It will keep its effect even after washing the items/them getting wet. NEVER apply permethrin directly to the skin. Treat your items, and let them dry completely before using.

To learn more about effective repellents, see the EPA site: http://cfpub.epa.gov/oppref/insect/index.cfm

Protect your pets, protect yourself

You should also protect your pets. If you have pets who go outside, and/or live in Northern latitudes in particular, keep up with their flea and tick prevention. Make them also wear a collar, and inspect them regularly for ticks.

Bathe them regularly as well, and try to avoid sleeping with them in order to lower your risk of being bitten by a tick hitchhiking on your pet. Discourage the children from sleeping with them or having them up on the furniture, and don't let them lay down on the floor with the pets or in the pet's bed. Keep your pets well-groomed, especially if they are a long-haired breed. Keep the fur cut short on legs and underbelly. Inspect these areas, plus the ears, chest and muzzle.

How to Remove Ticks From Yourself or Your Pet

It is essential to remove a tick correctly in case it is carrying the bacteria that trigger LD. The mouth parts can get lodged in the skin, if you are not careful, and as with bee venom, if you try to pluck off the tick with your fingers, you could be introducing even more poisonous substances into the body.

There are commercial tick removers on the market, http://amzn.to/2nBrjoV, but you really don't need to spend a lot of money on these items if you have a pair of fine-tipped tweezers in the house, http://amzn.to/2omYERP. The tweezers give more control and pose less risk from the tick.

You will need:
- Fine-tipped tweezers
- Rubbing alcohol
- A small disposable container, preferably with a cap.
- Sterile cotton
- a small magnifying glass if you have one
- Soap and warm water, or hand sanitizer if you are outdoors

Lay out your items on a clean surface, or a paper towel so you have everything ready.

To remove the tick:
Over the mouth of the small container, hold the tweezers and pour some of the rubbing alcohol over the tips to disinfect them.

Keep pouring until there is enough alcohol in the small container to submerge a tick completely.

Using the magnifying glass, if you have one, to see well, and the fine-tipped tweezers, focus your attention on the area where the tick's mouth parts are in the skin.

Aim the tweezer tips to try to grasp the tick as close as possible to the skin's surface. You don't want to squash the tick's head or body.

Squeeze the tweezers closed so you have a firm grip on the mouth part. Pull straight upwards out of your skin using a firm, steady movement. Do not yank, jerk or twist.

Place the tick in the rubbing alcohol. Swish around the tweezers to help disinfect them. Put a lid on the container if you have one and dispose of it. If there is no lid, flush it down the nearest toilet.

Wash your hands and the area of the tick bite carefully. If you don't have running water, use hand sanitizer and some alcohol on the cotton to clean the area of the bite.

If you were not able to get all of the mouth parts easily the first time, use the pointed tips to see if you can pull them out. If you can't, wash the area, use alcohol on a cotton ball, and leave it to heal. Don't try digging down for it as that can cause more than just the LD infection.

For a pet, part the fur as best you can so you can see the mouth parts. If the thought of dealing with the tick grosses you out, stick them under the shower or garden hose, aiming it at the spot with the tick. It will usually detach. Kill it if you can.

If you love the great outdoors or live outside the city and have pets, be vigilant about ticks and tick removal to keep you and your family as safe as possible from tick bites, which can cause a range of nasty illnesses, not just LD.

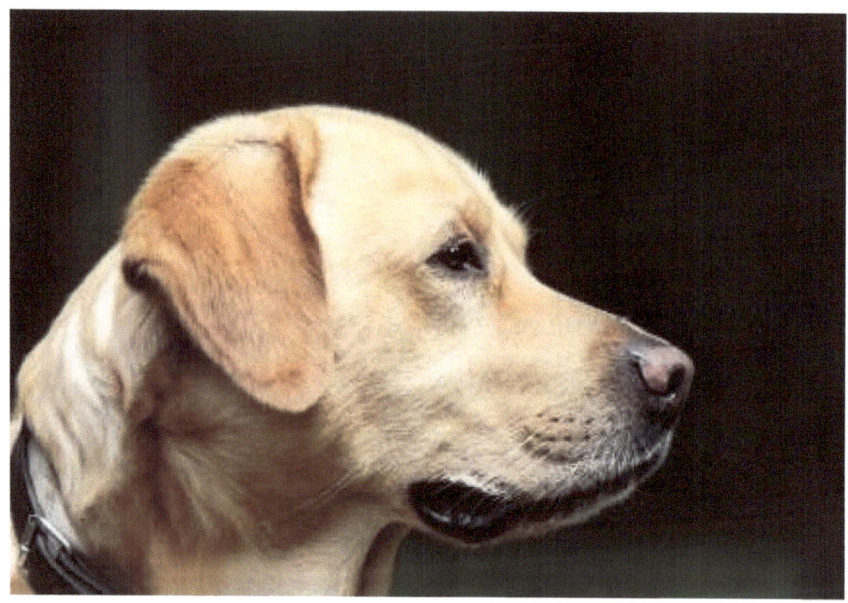

The Importance of Early Detection for Effective Treatment

Early detection is essential for effective treatment of Lyme disease. The trouble is that only about 70% to 80% of those who contract it show the telltale bullseye rash that can distinguish Lyme from other medical conditions.

Early stage Lyme disease

Early stage Lyme presents some diagnostic difficulties because of many of its symptoms are similar to common illnesses such as the flu, aches and pains, tiredness from overexertion, and so on. Up until recently, a large percentage of the medical community in the US didn't believe that Lyme even existed. They thought it might be other issues such as fibromyalgia, some sort of autoimmune 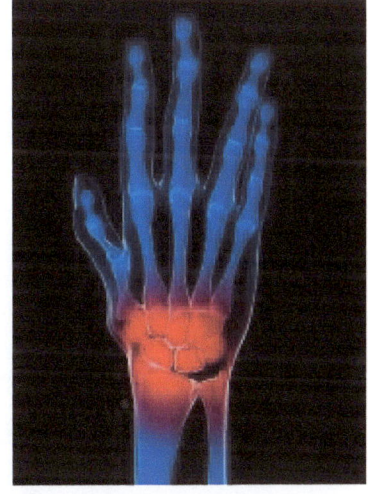 disorder like multiple sclerosis (MS) or rheumatoid arthritis (RA), chronic fatigue syndrome (CFS), or it being 'all in the patient's head.'

Fortunately, most doctors are now a lot better informed about Lyme disease, so presenting to the doctor with the typical symptoms, but also taking a full medical history, can help determine earlier than ever whether or not the person has Lyme disease.

A precise medical history

Doctors in the Northeast and Northwestern US should ask about the person's hobbies and where they have been recently, such as hiking or camping. They should also ask whether there are pets in the house such as cats or dogs, and whether they go out into wooded areas.

They should also be asked if they saw a tick attached to them, and whether or not they tried to remove it. If they tried to remove it, did they do so successfully, or might there still be tick mouth parts embedded in the skin.

If the person lives in an area where Lyme is common, or they have seen a tick, the doctor will likely not wait to start the patient on antibiotics. This is because the bacteria is a spirochete, which looks like a corkscrew. Because of its shape, it can insert itself into tissue and be very difficult to eradicate.

Effective treatment for Lyme

Depending on severity of symptoms and patient allergies, doctors may recommend one or more antibiotics to try to prevent the bacteria from spreading. The antibiotics might be intravenous, by mouth, or both. Oral antibiotic treatments will usually last 2 to 4 weeks. The whole course should be taken even if the patient starts to feel better, and they should go for follow up tests with the doctor to determine the level of bacterial activity in the blood.

Advanced Lyme disease

Prompt treatment is the best hope of success in eradicating Lyme before it can do serious damage. However, if the disease remains untreated, it can result in serious health issues, including:

- **Neurological disorders** - These include headache, stiff neck, nerve pain, 'brain fog', and in some cases facial nerve paralysis, commonly referred to as Bell's palsy. The cognitive decline that results from untreated Lyme has been mistaken for dementia and Alzheimer's disease.

- **Heart problems** - Lyme carditis is an infection of the heart muscle which can lead to a slow or fast heart rate, or irregular beats.

- **Eye issues** - Lyme can cause a range of vision problems, from pink eye (conjunctivitis) and blurred vision, to dry eye and more serious irritations.

- **Rheumatological issues** - The pain in bones in joints has been compared to them feeling as though they are on fire. Along with muscle aches and fatigue, it is often mistaken for fibromyalgia and other rheumatic conditions.

Since the complications of Lyme disease can lead to a severely diminished quality of life, if you suspect you have Lyme, have it checked out as soon as possible to get the treatment you need.

Myths and Misconceptions

There are a lot of myths and misconceptions about Lyme disease. This is because until recently many doctors actually doubted the condition even existed, despite more than 100 years of documented cases worldwide, and 40 years of medical history in the US.

Not every doctor is Lyme-savvy, so if you think you have Lyme disease, it is important to distinguish fact from fiction in order to prevent Lyme disease, or to get the most effective treatment if you do happen to contract it.

Here are some of the most common myths and misconceptions about Lyme, and the true facts.

MYTH: You can get Lyme in all 50 states in the US.
Fact. Lyme has only been contracted in 14 states thus far. However, travelers have picked up Lyme while visiting these 14 states. In 2015, 95% of confirmed Lyme disease cases were reported from:
- Connecticut
- Delaware
- Maine
- Maryland
- Massachusetts
- Minnesota
- New Hampshire
- New Jersey
- New York
- Pennsylvania
- Rhode Island

- Vermont
- Virginia
- Wisconsin

Some pockets have been reported in the Pacific Northwest, such as around the San Francisco Bay area, where it tends to be cool most of the year.

Myth: Lyme ticks love hot weather.
Fact. Lyme carrying ticks prefer cooler weather in northern latitudes.

MYTH: You can only catch Lyme in the US.
Fact. Lyme is present in 80 countries around the world. If there are deer, there is a danger of Lyme being transmitted by a tick.

MYTH: You can catch Lyme from any tick that bites you.
Fact. Only 3 ticks are known to carry Lyme:
- The black-legged tick, also known as the deer tick
- The Western black-legged tick
- The Lone Star tick

It is important to note that ticks can carry a range of tickborne diseases apart from or in addition to Lyme disease.

MYTH: All my strange symptoms are caused by Lyme disease.
Fact. About one-third of all Lyme patients have a co-infection, that is, an additional infection from the tick bite. Ticks feed on mammals, reptiles and amphibians. In doing so, they can become the vector or source of a range of illnesses.

In those with co-infections, about one-third have babesiosis, a parasitical infection of the red blood cells that is similar to malaria. The symptoms are the same as Lyme, but patients might also experience high fever, chills, and drenching sweats.

One-third with co-infections might have bartonella, also known as cat scratch fever because it is commonly carried by cat. The symptoms are similar to Lyme, but may also include:

- Poor appetite
- An unusual streaked rash that resembles "stretch marks" from pregnancy
- Swollen glands in the neck and under the arms
- Neurological symptoms such as:
- blurred vision
- numbness in the hands and feet
- memory loss
- balance problems
- trouble walking and
- tremors such as with Parkinson's disease.

If your doctor tells you that your symptoms are unusual for a person with Lyme, ask them to check for co-infection. Fortunately, a course of one or more antibiotics can usually clear up Lyme as well as other co-infections, but the more prompt the treatment, the better.

MYTH: You can't contract Lyme disease in the winter. **Fact.** While it is true that most cases are reported in the spring and summer months, the deer tick can survive even in very cold climates.

Those who enjoy being outdoors in the winter and who let their pets out should still be vigilant about tick bites.

MYTH: Everyone with Lyme disease gets a bullseye rash.
Fact. Only about 70& to 80% of Lyme patients get the bullseye rash. Therefore, it is important to be alert about Lyme symptoms. If you go walking in a wooded area or one with tall grass and then start to feel as though you have the flu a couple of days later, or find an attached tick on your body, it would be wise to suspect Lyme disease even if you have no rash.

MYTH: If the test is negative, you don't have Lyme.
Fact. The current standard blood test, known as ELISA, is not always accurate. Its accuracy increases the longer a person has had Lyme, because there will be a larger number of antibodies against the Lyme bacteria Borrelia burgdorferi in the blood stream. At the moment, the test is only about 60% accurate.

MYTH: If the test is positive, you do have Lyme.
Fact. The ELISA test can also have a false positive, that is, register that you have Lyme, even though you might have another health issue. This is because you might have been exposed to Lyme in the past. You might have had symptoms and been cured, or it may have been present in your blood stream but lain dormant.

A false positive can be a dangerous thing because the doctor will treat you for Lyme, but not for the condition you actually have.

MYTH: Antibiotics cure all cases of Lyme disease.
Fact. While it is true that early treatment with antibiotics can be effective against Lyme, the earlier it is caught, the better. Delays in treatment can result in long-term symptoms, which are referred to as chronic Lyme disease. (CLD). There are around 3 million Americans with Lyme disease, with 300,000 new cases being reported each year. On average, about 20% of patients will develop CLD even after antibiotic treatment.

MYTH: Chronic Lyme Disease (CLD) will go away on its own over time.
Fact: There is no evidence to suggest Lyme disease clears the body without treatment. In fact, the opposite is true. The longer it remains untreated, the more damage it can cause to the body.

MYTH: Lyme disease isn't that serious.
Fact. Untreated Lyme disease can be fatal. Lyme carditis can affect the heart and lead to sudden cardiac arrest and death.

MYTH: There's no reason to treat Chronic Lyme Disease, because once you have it, there isn't much chance of getting any better.
Fact. This is a dangerous myth that causes a great deal of misery for people who could improve their quality of life if they were more proactive. A balanced diet, exercise, antibiotic treatment as needed, and complementary therapies can all help relieve the more miserable symptoms of CLD.

Myth: If the person doesn't look sick, they can't have Lyme disease.

Fact. Many illnesses and disabilities are invisible. In the case of Lyme, it's possible to be very ill and outwardly look fine.

Typical symptoms of CLD include:

- fatigue
- low energy levels
- memory loss
- brain 'fog'
- cognitive impairment to the point where people think it is dementia
- muscle ache
- joint pain
- heart issues

MYTH: Once a person gets treatment for Lyme, they will start to feel better right away.

Fact. The worst thing about Lyme can often be the treatment. This is because the bacteria release toxins as they die off, causing an extreme reaction in the body termed an inflammatory response. This leads to ache, pains, flu-like symptoms, and the sensation that their bones and joints are on fire. Flushing out the toxins by drinking lots of water with lemon juice can help, but in general, the patient just has to ride it out until the episode subsides.

These episodes are called Jarisch-Herxheimer Reactions, or Herxes for short. They can be potentially dangerous due to them triggering severe neurological symptoms, so it is important to work closely with your doctor to minimize risk and misery.

MYTH: The only effective way to treat Lyme is with antibiotics.

Fact. While it is true that antibiotics are the foundation for effective treatment, complementary therapies can help, such as acupressure, massage and aromatherapy.

Final Thoughts

Lyme disease can range in impact on your health between a mild inconvenience to a debilitating disease similar to arthritis. It can also affect the heart and brain. In addition, it can affect the nerves, leading to paralysis.

While there are effective treatments to relieve the symptoms of LD, prevention is really the best way to help your health. Watch out if you are heading into the wild, and take precautions so you don't get bitten by any disease-bearing bugs, including ticks.

An ounce of prevention is worth a pound of cure when it comes to the misery of Lyme disease.

Stay safe, and stay well!

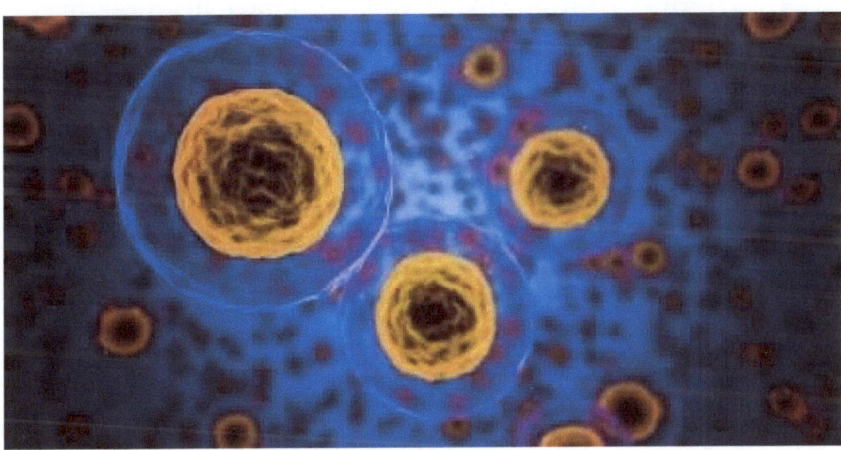

Lyme Disease Symptoms Checklist

These symptoms may appear 3 to 30 days after a tick bite.

The most important thing to know about Lyme Disease is the symptoms to watch out for. Ticks are very small, and their bite isn't always that obvious. If you live in Northern latitudes and/or have pets that spend a lot of time outside, and you develop any of the following symptoms, it could be a sign of Lyme disease infection:

Early Signs and Symptoms of Lyme Disease (Acute Lyme Disease)

Flu-like symptoms, which can include:
- Fever
- Chills
- Headache
- Tiredness/fatigue even when you have been resting and not been active
- Muscle pain
- Aching joint aches
- Swollen lymph nodes, such as in the neck
- Bullseye rash-this occurs in around 80% of cases. The rash will gradually expand its diameter over time. It can appear on any limb. It is not usually painful or itchy.
- Bell's palsy-paralysis of a facial nerve on one side of the face, causing a drooping appearance and problems speaking; often mistaken for stroke
- Lyme titer activity in the blood, though up to 50% can be false positive results

Chronic Lyme Disease

These Signs and Symptoms can manifest days to months after the tick bite and last for months or years.

In most cases, the treatment for acute Lyme is antibiotics, intravenous and/or oral. Antibiotic treatment is usually successful, but some people have lingering symptoms after the acute phase. This is termed Chronic Lyme Disease and can be characterized by one or more of the following:

- Flu-like symptoms
- Severe headaches/migraine
- Neck stiffness
- Inflammation of the brain and spinal cord, sometimes mistaken for meningitis
- Problems with short-term memory, 'brain fog'
- Spirochete activity in the blood stream (corkscrew-like bacteria
- Lyme titer activity in the blood stream
- Bullseye rashes appearing on more than one area of the body
- Arthritis with severe joint pain and swelling, particularly in the large joints.
- A feeling that your 'bones are on fire'
- Bell's palsy, temporary or permanent
- Muscle aches and pains that come and go
- Numbness, sharp pains, or tingling in the limbs, hands or feet
- Heart palpitations, or an irregular heart beat (Lyme carditis)
- Episodes of dizziness or shortness of breath, fainting
- Nerve pain in one area, or throughout the body
- Upset stomach from the antibiotics

- More severe symptoms after taking antibiotics, due to the spirochetes releasing toxins into the body. Severe head and stomach aches can be common.

Symptoms are most severe when rash is present, less severe when no rash is seen.

Other Relevant Books by This Author

If you would like to read more relevant books about this topic, here is a list of the CreateSpace links, titles and descriptions from this author:

https://www.createspace.com/6794823

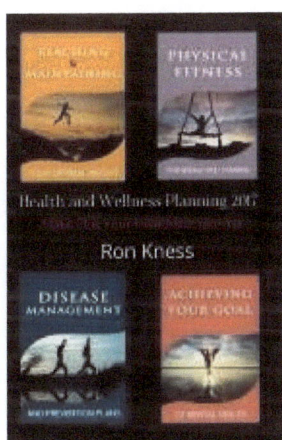

Health and Wellness Planning - 2017: 4 Reports to Help Make This Your Healthiest Year Yet

Your doctor is a valuable resource when it comes to your health and fitness concerns. However, many people don't know how to talk to their doctors.

After some visits, you might even leave the doctor's office with more questions than answers. Maybe you feel that you don't have a chance during your appointment to say what's really on your mind.

Talking to your doctor is very important before you begin any new fitness and exercise regimen, especially if you have been quite sedentary up until now. Here are some tips to help you prepare so you can leave your next appointment with the best answers possible.

- Bring up the topic of fitness and exercise yourself. If you wait for your doctor to mention it, the subject may not come up. Some doctors are reluctant to bring up fitness and exercise because they don't want to hurt their patients' feelings.

- Prepare your questions ahead of time. Your doctor has budgeted only a certain amount of time to spend with you. You can make your appointment run more quickly and smoothly by writing down your questions ahead of time. When your appointment starts, let your doctor know that you have a list of questions. That will indicate to your doctor that you are seeking particular information and they will usually give you the opportunity to work your way through the list.

- Ask about what kinds of exercise you should be doing. Your doctor will know your medical history and will know if certain types of exercise would be unwise for you to try. They may be concerned about you getting injured. As well, if you have any medical conditions or are taking any medications, that might affect your ability to do certain exercises.

- Ask about your resting heart rate and what your target heart rate should be. Your doctor can explain these to you. Your doctor will be able to tell you what your target heart rate should be based on your age and medical condition. He or she can also show you how to easily calculate your heart rate.

- If you want to lose weight, this is a good opportunity to discuss a reasonable weight-loss goal with your doctor. He or she will be able to tell you what a realistic weight loss would be for your condition. They can also help you determine your ideal weight.

- Ask about diet and nutrition. Your doctor can tell you how many calories you should be eating each day to stay healthy and may recommend certain foods to improve and maintain your health.

- Take notes. While your doctor is speaking, take notes of their answers. With so much information being thrown at you, it will be impossible to remember all of it. You may also want to bring along a friend to ask any questions you didn't think of and to help remind you of important details after you leave.

Your doctor is an important partner in your health care. By taking this advice, you will be able to start a meaningful conversation with your doctor and gain helpful information.

In this book are four reports that after reading may help you better plan your next trip with your doctor in regard to health and fitness:
• Achieving Your Goal of Mental Health
• Disease Management and Prevention Plans
• Physical Fitness for Energy and Stamina
• Reaching and Maintaining Your Optimal Weight

These 4 reports will not only help you improve your health and wellness, but also serve to spur meaningful conversations with your doctor.

https://www.createspace.com/6433160

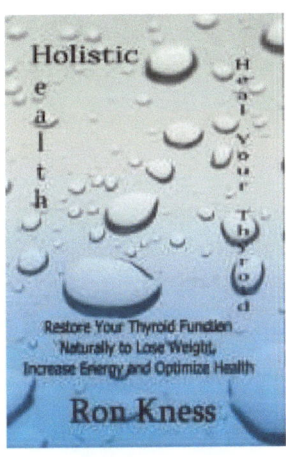

Heal Your Thyroid: Restore Your Thyroid Function Naturally to Lose Weight, Increase Energy and Optimize Health

The thyroid is a gland that is responsible for regulating many of your bodily functions and if it isn't functioning properly, you will experience a variety of symptoms that can impact your life in unfavorable ways.

The problem is that diagnosing a thyroid disorder can be difficult because the symptoms can be vague and attributed to many different things. Because of this, millions of people wake up every day with thyroid issues without even knowing it.

- Do you constantly feel so fatigued that you barely have the energy to brush your teeth?

- Do you find that there is more hair than usual ending up in your brush or shower drain?

- Are you gaining weight or just not losing no matter how much you try to adapt a healthy lifestyle?

- Do you often feel cold or have sensitivity to cold temperatures?

- Do you have constant brain fog or memory issues?

- Do you have dry eyes?

Well most of us experience these things at various times and because we simply assume that age is catching up with us or that we are not exercising as frequently as we should or that we are not getting enough sleep…we just chalk them up to something we have to live with and don't pursue any medical follow-up.

Many times it is an under-performing thyroid that is causing problems. With the proper nutrition, exercise and some lifestyle changes, you can heal your thyroid. They are all things you should be doing anyway, so what do you have to lose?

https://www.createspace.com/6558396

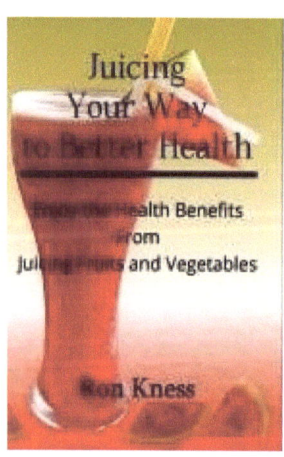

Juicing Your Way to Better Health: Enjoy the Health Benefits from Juicing Fruits and Vegetables

Whether it is just a fad or a trend that is here to stay, juicing is extremely popular among health conscious individuals. As more and more people experience the amazing results associated with this healthy lifestyle choice, its popularity is expected to grow.

Without question, juicing can be incorporated into your daily life to increase your overall health and vitality. By increasing your daily intake of healthy fruits and vegetables, you'll be giving your body the essential building blocks it needs. To get the most benefit out of juicing, you'll want to educate yourself on some of the basics before you get started.

In my book "Juicing Your Way to Better Health", you'll find a wealth of information on juicing.

If you are new to juicing, you may find the process to be a bit of a hassle. However, once you start to see and experience the many benefits associated with juicing, you may wonder how you ever got along without it. So commit to testing out your new lifestyle using juice from fruits and vegetables for at least several weeks before deciding if it is for you or not.

Once you start to reap the health benefits, you'll be hooked on juicing. Get started now!

About the Author

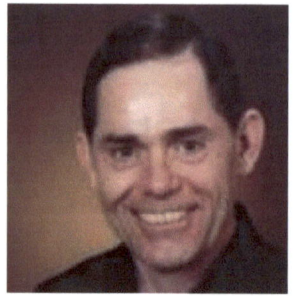

I have published over 125 books on Amazon for Kindle, CreateSpace and other publishing platforms.

While most of my books are on health and fitness in general, as I age (now 65) at the time of this writing) my topics of interest are geared toward aging baby boomers and older. Besides my own writing, I also ghostwrite ebooks, books, reports, articles, blogs and do Kindle conversions for clients on a variety of topics.

Today my wife and I are retired from our careers and live in Gold Canyon, AZ. I now write as a retirement business where you'll find me happily sitting in my office typing away on my laptop as I work on my next book or ghostwriting project . . . that is if we are not traveling on a cruise ship - our new-found mode of travel.

www.ingramcontent.com/pod-product-compliance
Lightning Source LLC
Chambersburg PA
CBHW050817290526
45792CB00001B/148